Ha, I Laugh in the Face of Cancer

SUSAN LIBERTY HALL

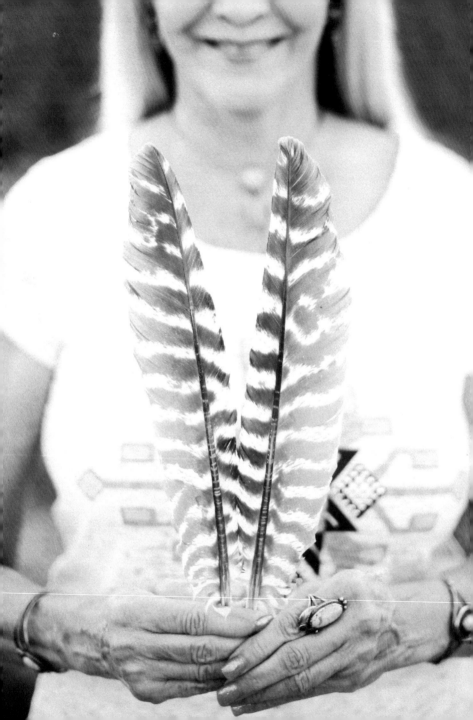

Ha, I Laugh in the Face of Cancer

By Susan Liberty Hall

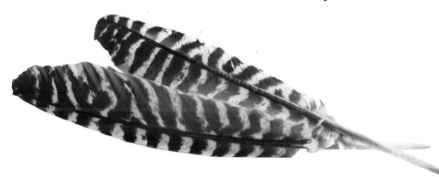

Also By Susan Liberty Hall
Scented Adventures of
The Bouquet Sisters in Fairyland

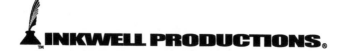

ISBN: 978-1-939625-67-0

Library of Congress Control Number: 2014900204

Published by Inkwell Productions
10869 N Scottsdale Road #103-128
Scottsdale, AZ 85254-5280
Phone: 480-315-3781
E-mail: info@inkwellproductions.com
www.inkwellproductions.com

Printed in the United States of America.

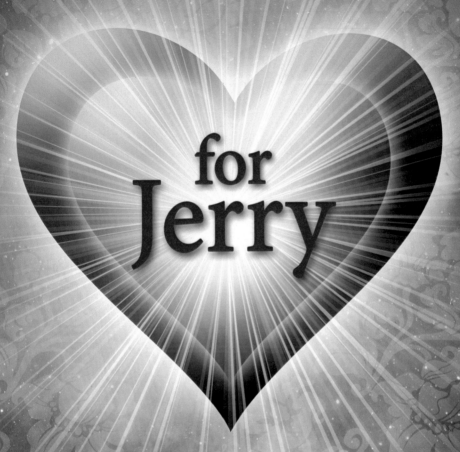

for Jerry

This book is dedicated to my Beloved Brother, Jerry Buss, whose glorious love is imprinted forever upon everyone he knew.

Acknowledgment

I would like to introduce to my readers the most
amazing Cancer Protocol I have ever encountered.
It is the American Indian Herbal Remedy,
Two Feathers Healing Formula. As you read my little
book you will discover how I was able to overcome
the dreaded Cancer with a simple Protocol.

With that in mind, I would like to honor Robert Roy
and the American Indian Medicine Men and Women
who have had the Wisdom to understand the
healing ability of the Earth Mother for all People.

You have saved my life, and our work has just begun.
I offer you my profound gratitude.

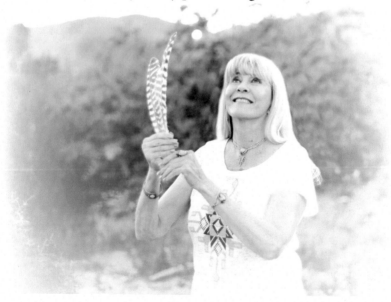

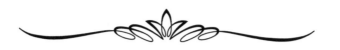

Contents

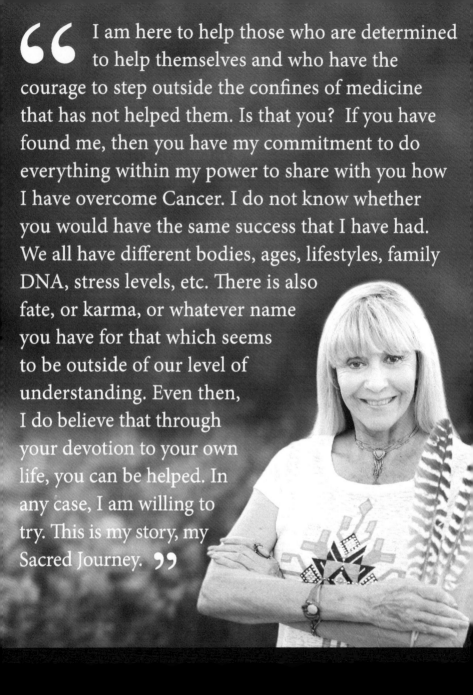

" I am here to help those who are determined to help themselves and who have the courage to step outside the confines of medicine that has not helped them. Is that you? If you have found me, then you have my commitment to do everything within my power to share with you how I have overcome Cancer. I do not know whether you would have the same success that I have had. We all have different bodies, ages, lifestyles, family DNA, stress levels, etc. There is also fate, or karma, or whatever name you have for that which seems to be outside of our level of understanding. Even then, I do believe that through your devotion to your own life, you can be helped. In any case, I am willing to try. This is my story, my Sacred Journey. **"**

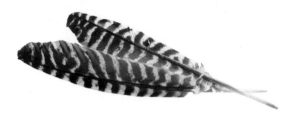

Introduction

If You Look for the Cure Where It Is Not, You Will Not Find It There

They say that laughter is the best medicine. If that is true, then it is important that we use laughter to lessen the fear and horror of hearing those terrible words, "You have Cancer." However, I was not laughing when my mom died of Cancer, nor when my brother died of Cancer.

This is the dreaded disease, the death sentence, that brings images of gaunt and yellow faces, bald and frightened looking ... and not knowing what to do or where to go, or how to escape their situation.

Most people believe that the brilliant Medical Doctors, the renowned researchers, and heavily funded Research programs surely have the best answers. Or, do they???

"Run for the Cure," and so many charities and fund raisers have raised hundreds of millions of dollars, or even much more, year after year. IF YOU LOOK FOR THE CURE WHERE IT IS NOT, YOU WILL NOT FIND IT THERE! No matter how far you run or how many millions of people may run.

What would it look like if all of those funds were channeled into why people get Cancer in the first place and how to avoid it altogether? What significant improvement has there been in conventional Cancer treatments in the last 50 years or more? What is the actual success rate for those treatments? I have recently read it is about 3%. Just do the research for yourself before you make your decision.

If you believe, however, that your best chance is where the money, research, and medical practice is, then follow their program and give it your very best. I do not want to influence you against conventional medicine if that is your choice. I do not want to confuse you with the facts and overwhelming evidence and personal testimonials in the thousands to support the validity of the Two Feathers Healing Formula, starting with me.

The healing modality that will be revealed to you in this little book is simple and empowering, with everything that you need to make a conscious, well-informed decision for your success without fear and without financial devastation to you. This modality would also save the terrible financial burden upon our hospitals, clinics, hospice, and insurance and Medicare agencies as well.

How would that impact the cost of our insurance, if there were no Chemo-so-called-Therapy, Radiation, never-ending surgeries, nor the hospitalization that it entails, and creates? These are money makers for the Morticians, but I do not choose to support them through Cancer deaths! This treatment is for you as an individual and offers you the opportunity to heal yourself, and could also miraculously heal the outrageous costs associated with each and every Cancer case! Don't forget, either, about the devastation to your family members, because they suffer right along with you.

Whatever course you choose, you have my purest and sweetest blessing, and all of you are in my daily prayers. It would be appropriate to remember, as well, the Biblical advice: "Physician, heal thyself."

But if you have seen the evidence of broken lives and death and devastation by those who have not been helped by conventional medicine, then you are the ones I wish to reach. If you say, "Oh, I can't do anything that isn't covered by my insurance, " or "I can't do anything that my Doctor doesn't suggest," then this is definitely not for you. If you do tell your Doctor that you are doing an American Indian Medicine Men and Women Healing Formula, instead of Surgery, Chemo and Radiation treatments, they may not allow you to continue as their patient. I know, because it happened to me. My Doctor would not allow me to continue as his patient when I refused to do the Mastectomy, Chemo, and Radiation.

If you wish to read on, then please know that I am not a medical expert; I have no medical knowledge or understanding. I am simply someone who has overcome Cancer, and I am Cancer-free. I hope you will realize the importance of not making me responsible for your own choices. Please accept responsibility for your own illness and be responsible for your own healing. Then, I will be devoted to helping you.

We each must earn our own healing. If you are looking for a magic pill that your Doctor can give you, that requires nothing of you, then don't look to me for help. If you are not willing to honestly change your lifestyle, to do the nutrition, exercise, supplements, emotional issues, prayers, and devotion necessary to win your healing, then just stay with your Doctor.

I know that all Doctors must take the Hippocratic Oath, to "First do no harm." So it is unbelievable to me that they are prescribing all of these drugs and procedures that have a warning list a mile long, creating a disclaimer from any responsibility. If you get any of the diseases that the prescription or procedure may very well develop in your body, then, oh well! There will be no trouble for the Pharmaceuticals, AMA, FDA, your Doctor, Hospital, or anyone else. The attorneys will be there to make a fortune, but it is you who will pay the ultimate price.

Whatever happened to "common sense"? If you have a disease and are taking a prescription drug for that disease that has a possible consequence like Cancer, Diabetes, Liver failure, or "some fatal events have been reported" (fatal events???), that means you could die from the treatment. The list goes on and on... so why would you take it in the first place?

I have a good friend who is very confident about conventional medicine, and she was questioning me about how I know I am Cancer-free. I explained to her about the AMAS blood test that determines that for me. She was skeptical and told me that I could go to a Doctor who would give me a test that could "really" determine whether I was Cancer-free. She said it was very easy. All I had to do was drink a glass or two of radioactive material, then take a CAT Scan. How could I drink a poison that we all know causes Cancer to determine whether I *have* Cancer? If I didn't have Cancer before the test, I could very well develop it after the test.

I do not understand this kind of reasoning; not by individuals and especially not by Doctors. I do not understand how we, as a people of flesh and blood, are so willing to ingest or inject ourselves with known Carcinogens just because the Doctors tell us to!

I am very grateful to the Medical Doctors, and especially the Naturopathic Doctors, for all of the good that they do. Truly, they are heroes, and I honor them for helping people with accidents and all kinds of illness where they are "truly helpful" and not harmful. My concern is the use of dangerous drugs and pharmaceuticals that they promote. If there is no assistance for the patient to correct his own lifestyle that has created this illness, then there can be no real Victory. Drugs alone will never bring the healing of the body, and the patient must take his place as the determiner of his own fate.

Doctors receive their Medical education at Universities. Who is it that funds their education? Is it the Pharmaceutical Companies that have a platform to deliver their drugs through the Doctors that they are educating? If it has a "patent," as most drugs do, then it is easy to understand that you will pay a fortune to get it, the Insurance and Medicare programs will pay to the point of bankrupting the system, and that will, in turn, impact our Beloved Country as well.

But a natural product that God has made, in its natural state, cannot be patented. It is freely available to all. Is it time to rethink our Medical system and Pharmaceutical dependence?

No matter how much it costs to care for a Cancer patient, if the result is failure and hell and misery, then it is insult added to injury!

I am here to help those who are determined to help themselves and who have the courage to step outside the confines of medicine that has not helped them. Is that you? If you have found me, then you have my commitment to do everything within my power to share with you how I have overcome Cancer.

I do not know whether you would have the same success that I have had. We all have different bodies, ages, lifestyles, family DNA, stress levels, etc. There is also fate, or karma, or whatever name you have for that which seems to be outside of our level of understanding. Even then, I do believe that through your devotion to your own life, you can be helped. In any case, I am willing to try. This is my story, my Sacred Journey.

I am a 68-year-old grandmother, very healthy and active, running my own Young Living Essential Oils business; Author of a children's book, *Scented Adventures of The Bouquet Sisters in Fairyland*; and just enjoying the fruits of my life's labors, when suddenly, in April 2012, I was diagnosed with Cancer in my right breast.

At this same time, my beloved brother, Jerry Buss, was also diagnosed with Cancer. He called to tell me the news and about his decision to begin aggressive Chemo and Radiation treatments immediately, to be followed by a Surgery to remove the tumor that had been discovered in his abdomen. I chose not to tell him that I also had Cancer, and I knew that the time would come when I could share that fact with him, but at a more appropriate time.

Cancer was not new to our family. Our mother Jessie was diagnosed with colon Cancer when she was only 61 years old. I was living in Japan with my son, enjoying my life, and I was devastated by the bad news. Jerry asked me to come home to take care of our mom. I left Tokyo the next day, not realizing that I would never return to the beautiful apartment that I had in Akasaka and that I would leave my life in Japan behind me forever.

None of that mattered now. The only issue was helping mom. I moved in with her and was with her constantly for the next nine months of her life. She began a rigorous regimen of Chemo, and I dutifully drove her to her appointments where the Doctor would deliver the horrifying treatment. She was terrified. The treatments were very painful, and each treatment was worse than the one before. Her veins did not receive the poison well, as her body tried to resist that which was never meant to be injected or ingested into human bodies.

She would vomit, and she could not eat. She had no appetite, and she could not sleep. There was nothing that I could do to help, except to love her, and be with her on her journey—but this was not a Sacred Journey.

I prayed every day for mercy and some kind of solution. I did some study about the Chemo treatment, and I was very upset to understand that the Chemo killed the Cancer, but at the same time it also was killing the patient. It was, in my opinion, a gambler's bet on what would die first: the Cancer or the patient? I did not like the odds.

She tried to do everything the Doctor said. When she could not eat, I asked her to let me help her with nutrition. I suggested some vitamin pills and nutritious foods. She had no interest whatsoever in my suggestions. I was looking into pure, organic foods without pesticides and chemical poisonings. She had no faith in my ideas at all. She would not even take a vitamin pill unless the Doctor told her to do so.

I asked her Doctor whether he would tell her of the importance of nutrition and supplementation to help her condition. He laughed at me, however, and told her in my presence that it was not necessary to take supplements and that she could eat anything she wanted. He suggested cakes, cookies, pies, anything that she wanted, and that it was not important or necessary to take vitamins or to be concerned with nutrition. Dr. God had spoken, and I was dismissed.

This began my education about the conventional Doctor's lack of interest in the health and care of the human body, the issues of prevention and the building up of the body's immune system so that the Cancer could be fought off. NO. None of this was important then, in 1978, and none of that is important today, in 2013, because I received the same exact information when my beloved brother Jerry had his Cancer treatments.

My mother suffered so much. Every day was a misery. Pain, grief, worry, and fear were her only emotions. She was losing weight at an alarming rate, and she would seldom leave her bed. When she did leave her bed, she could hardly walk without assistance, and in the night I caught her actually crawling to the bathroom. Then I started sleeping at the foot of her bed so that I could help her. She did not want visitors, not relatives or friends, because she was embarrassed by her appearance. It is true; she looked terrible. Her hair was falling out, and she was jaundiced—even the whites of her eyes were yellow. I suffered along with her. There is something to be said about quality of life and not just quantity of misery.

After a few agonizing months, my mother was put into the hospital, and exploratory surgery was done to look at the Cancer. It had metastasized, and there was nothing the Doctors could do, except to sew her up and tell us the verdict: IMMINENT DEATH! So much for Chemo treatments!

Speaking of Chemo, I have heard that there is a prestigious medical study out of Poland that has revealed that Chemo actually *causes* Cancer. While it may be true that it also kills Cancer, does it make sense to take it if it actually also causes Cancer? I believe that soon it will be considered barbaric to treat Cancer with Chemo and Radiation. It will be looked upon as very foolish, especially since it destroys the Immune System that is necessary to fight the Cancer.

Look at the vicious circle. You take Chemo and Radiation to kill the Cancer. They destroy the immune system, and it creates more Cancer. In any case, please do not accept my understanding of this. Do your own research; find out for yourself, and do not give your power of choice away to anyone else! It is your life—no one has as great an interest in your survival than you do.

For your consideration, here is another insight I have learned. Our God has given us a way to deal with Cancer. If you eat organic fruits and vegetables—some of them raw and in the natural state, as God provided for us—your body can fight Cancer. But, if you are eating fruits, as an example, that have been treated with antifungal chemicals, then the plant loses its original blueprint, or understanding, about how to create its own antifungal properties. This means it cannot help fight the fungus in your body.

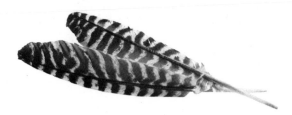

Chapter 1
Cancer Is a Fungus — and It Is Curable

Some amazing researchers believe that Cancer is caused by parasites or fungus: the work done by Hulda Clark, *The Cure for all Cancers*,[1] "Cancer Is a Fungus—and It Is Curable" by David Icke,[2] and more recently, Tullio Simoncini's work with Sodium Bicarbonate Therapy.[3] Dr. Simoncini's work uses a simple household compound. He was inspired to find a different approach for treating Cancer in view of the horrors he had witnessed with the children who were in the hospital receiving Chemo and Radiation treatments. It was so devastating that he determined to find another way, and he did; however, this ended him up in prison for his great humanitarian efforts! Also look at the work of Jim Humble: his Sodium Chlorite and Citric Acid solution, his book *The Miracle Mineral Solution of the 21st Century*,[4] and his Sodium Chlorite Water Purification Drops product.[5] These are just a few of some very promising, inexpensive, nontoxic ways to help anyone with Cancer. This is an education for the masses whose time has come. They can't put *everyone* in jail, can they? They did put Dr. Simoncini in jail. He has the courage and resolve to go ahead anyway!

But for me, there are only two ways that I have actually used and that I know without any doubt work for me. It is the Two Feathers Healing Formula[6] that I used faithfully, that took me from definitely having Breast Cancer to definitely **not** having Breast Cancer, together with the teachings of D. Gary Young and the Young Living Essential Oils, Supplements, and techniques[7] that have assisted my body to regain its strength and vitality, to restore my immune system, and to overcome Candida and the extreme stress that had compromised my body at this time. I used D. Gary Young's famous "Raindrop Technique" massage, using the oils to stimulate the immune system.

Now I will get back to my story, because it is my prayer that it will help you on your Sacred Journey, too.

My brother Jerry, who was very devoted to our mom, also suffered. He loved her so much. Even with all of his power and brilliance, his money and attainment, he also was powerless before the great enemy of Cancer. I remember he had just purchased the Los Angeles Lakers basketball team. He was at a press conference when the nurse in care of our mother alerted me that she was near death.

I called my brother immediately, and he left the press conference and came running to be with her. But it was too late. The nurse informed me that mom had died. When he arrived, he ran to her and picked her up in his arms, and I am a witness to the fact that one small tear fell from her eye and that she died in his arms. Yes, she had come back from the dead to be with him one last time. This is the great love my mother had for my brother. She was 62, and she would never enjoy the amazing success of her son Jerry.

This was the beginning of my search for an answer to Cancer. I understood that it could be hereditary and that I also could get this disease and so could my children and grandchildren. I devoted myself to this search and to natural, healthy living as a preventative for this insidious disease. I began a "Cancer file," and I would search for cures. The file was very thin, and I did not know whether I had found anything at all that could really heal Cancer.

The years passed, and I began my journey with Therapeutic Grade Essential Oils for health. It became the center of my life, and I was thrilled with my new discovery. I was using the Young Living Essential oils, and I was constantly amazed at my personal experiences, and testimonials of others. I listened to D. Gary Young about how to avoid Cancer and how to use nutrition and organic foods and supplements to help keep healthy and to strengthen the immune system.

I had not been well during this time. I had chronic fatigue, severe migraine headaches, and I was too ill to work. I had a devastating marriage that ended with my husband's suicide. There was a mountain of debt that he had incurred in his business. I had inherited his debts in Arizona, as it is a community property state. There were no funds or income of any kind. I had 35 cents when he died, the house was in foreclosure, and I had no telephone or even a car. He had taken all of my funds, and I was left destitute. But I had Jerry. I am so grateful that he opened the door of mercy for me and took care of the foreclosure, gave me a car, and helped me get back on my feet. My dear brother had the sweetest soul, and he loved me. I can never forget that he picked me up from the hell and misery into which I had fallen and that I was given another chance. Thank God!

But my health had been compromised. Even so, I began to get better using the Young Living Essential Oils, and I was able to overcome the agonizing migraines that had lasted for 2 or 3 weeks at a time. I began to exercise and to eat raw, organic foods. I followed the regimens of D. Gary Young and I knew that I had found the way to achieve health, despite the stress and terrible events of my marriage.

I had always suffered from chronic fatigue, although there was not a name for it in the early years. I had learned to live with it and had the hope that I could overcome it in my lifetime; however, now there was a new threat to my life: Breast Cancer! It surprised me, and I was in denial that I had it. I had ignored the two marble-size lumps that were growing on my right breast. I cannot explain why I would not go in to the Doctor for my regular checkup. This would have determined quickly that I had a problem. This is a wake-up call that I hope my readers will learn from my mistake and thus avoid this in your own lives. I do use the diagnostic tools of the Medical field but not the ones that are dangerous, like the PET Scan used to determine the presence of Cancer.

At this same time, my brother Jerry was also diagnosed with Cancer. I drove to Los Angeles from Phoenix to be with him for his first surgery, after he had had a series of Chemo treatments. I decided not to tell him of my illness until he had successfully had his surgery. When I did tell him, he was very concerned and told me that I would need to follow my Doctor's advice immediately, with a Mastectomy of the right breast and possibly the lymph nodes, if necessary, and of course Chemo and Radiation. I knew that I had to tell him that I could not do that! As he was worried about my choice, I was also worried about his.

Although he was so worried about my decision, he honored my choice, as he had always done. Meanwhile, I had a most important decision to make, and I thought very carefully about the program I would choose to fight this disease. My first choice would be that I would go to the NovaVita Spa/Clinic in Ecuador.[8] I knew that they used the Young Living Essential Oils there; however, I also knew the treatment would be very expensive. Like many people, Jerry did not realize the uses of Therapeutic Grade Essential Oils in medicine; he just thought they were like perfumes.

This was not the time for him to study the subject, as I understood he needed to focus on his own condition, and he was very sure that his best chance was conventional medicine. I was equally sure that my best chance was most certainly **NOT** conventional medicine.

I did not ask Jerry for the money to go to the clinic in Ecuador. He would have done anything for me, but he did not believe I could be saved by any means other than surgery, Chemo, and Radiation, as he was doing. Since I did not have the money to go to the amazing NovaVita Clinic, I was facing a real dilemma: what would I do to save my own life????

I turned to devotion and prayer, and I asked for the direction in which my God would have me go, and then I listened very intently. I stood up, walked over to my office file cabinet, opened the cabinet to "C," and removed a file marked "CANCER" that I had placed there maybe 20 years ago. I had forgotten all about it. I opened the file, and there was a picture of a man with a wound in his chest area, and next to the picture was another photo of 8 tumors that the man claimed had been released by using an American Indian herbal remedy called Two Feathers Healing Formula. I read the article and wondered, could it be true? How could that be? Would I be foolish to try this for myself? Would I be ridiculed by my family and friends?

I could not ignore the fact that I had asked in prayer and was given this answer. So, I immediately called the phone number and a man by the name of Robert Roy answered. I explained to him the condition that I had and asked to purchase a jar of the Two Feathers Healing Formula. I was determined to begin this regimen immediately. Robert Roy was so helpful. There was no charge for his assistance, and I knew that this was not just my own choice but also an answer to my prayer. Because of that, I was calm, and the fear I had felt before was now gone. Somehow, I felt certain that I had found the right answer for me and one that I could afford right now! This began my healing journey.

You may imagine the difficulty for me in having to tell my brother that I would be using an American Indian Medicine Men and Women herbal remedy and that I would be doing this by myself and not with the assistance of a Medical Doctor! In my opinion, Jerry was one of the most brilliant scientific minds in the world. He was the most intelligent, loving, amazing person I had ever known, and I was so blessed to be his sister, but, I could not go the way that he had chosen. I remember telling him, "I

Ha, I Laugh in the Face of Cancer

know that you are brilliant Jerry, but Nature is also brilliant!"
He respected my choice and was willing to support me in every
possible way.

So he began his treatments, and I began mine. My Doctor
sent me to a Breast Cancer Surgeon, and since it took 3 weeks to
get an appointment with her, I decided to begin the Two Feathers
Healing Formula protocol immediately. I learned that the Two
Feathers Healing Formula was over 100 years old and has been
used successfully for Cancer, tumors, and internal malignancies,
to cite only a few of its uses. It has also been used as a powerful
preventative remedy and detoxifier, for which it is used once or
twice a year.

I soon regretted the two biopsies that I had, being reminded
by several Naturopathic Doctors and other healers that it could
spread the Cancer. But how could I be sure that I had Cancer
without the biopsies? Like so many other people, I was frightened
by what I was told at the Breast Cancer Center and gave in to
having 3 biopsies, 2 of which were found to be cancerous.

Later, I would learn from Robert Roy, the distributor of the
Two Feathers Healing Formula that there is a simple blood test
called AMAS (Anti-Malignin Antibody in Serum)[9]—the antibody
test for Cancer—that could determine very accurately whether I
had Cancer and, if so, how advanced it was. Please see Chapter 5
for my own test results and more information on AMAS.)

I ordered the Two Feathers Healing Formula and began
taking it internally twice per day, in capsules, on April 5, 2012.
Fourteen days later, the first tumor had disappeared. It seemed to
have collapsed, and I could no longer see it or feel it. Then, 3 days

later, the second tumor also collapsed. Robert Roy explained to me that the Cancer was probably dead and that the evidence of this was that the tumors had detached from my living tissue. Now it was time to remove the dead tumors from my body.

At this time, I kept my original appointment with the Breast Surgeon that I had made 3 weeks before. I wanted to see and hear what she said and what she would suggest for me. She looked at my ultrasound, mammogram, and biopsy reports. She tried to feel the tumors that she could see in the report, but they were gone from her touch, and she had no explanation. I told her about the Two Feathers Healing Formula, and she said she was familiar with it. She called it "the black mud." She said it did not work and recommended an immediate Mastectomy for the right breast and possibly the removal of lymph nodes once I was in surgery. This was to be followed by Chemo and Radiation as well. I did not proceed any further with that option.

No Mastectomy for me, not now, not ever! I was a Playboy Bunny at the New Orleans Playboy Club in 1964. I also was a Playboy Bunny at the London Casino in 1967. I could not bear the thought that part of me would be sliced off, and then I would be irradiated and poisoned by Chemo. It was barbaric! It was a nightmare! I would take my chances with Nature instead.

I ordered 6 jars of the Two Feathers Healing Formula, so that I could get the lowest price, and used 5 of them over 5 months' time. This equates to a little over $100.00–$150.00 per month for 5 months to do the protocol. The amount of Two Feathers Healing Formula needed may vary for each individual, and this should be discussed with Robert Roy. I was doing this protocol by myself, without the help of a Doctor.

It was suggested by Robert Roy that I continue the internal use of the Two Feathers Healing Formula and that at the same time apply it to the location of the 2 tumors that had collapsed. I followed his suggestion. On May 12, just 5 weeks after I had begun using the Two Feathers Healing Formula, one of the tumors popped out and was released from the tumor site.

During that time, I could see the tumor emerging from my skin. I would reapply the Two Feathers Healing Formula every 3 days, and it was indeed very painful. I took pain pills to help me to continue the protocol. I collected the tumor that had just fallen out and put it in a specimen jar to use as evidence. The location where the tumor had come out had another tumor just under it that I could see, and it was obvious that I had more tumors that had to come out. I knew it would be tough, but not as tough as a Mastectomy, and not as sickening as Chemo and Radiation.

I was so grateful for my guidance, and for the choice that I had made. For the next 6 months I had an open wound at the tumor site. I never got an infection, and I used a simple spray of Colloidal Silver Water on the wound each day as Robert suggested. I also used my Young Living Essential Oils for Breast Cancer everyday: Frankincense, Myrtle, Sandalwood, and Tsuga.

Meanwhile, Jerry continued his protocol, and I went to Los Angeles every time he had a surgery or a procedure. He had at least 4 or 5 surgeries and 4 procedures to correct problems from the first surgery. It was never corrected. On the 27th day of his last Radiation treatment, I was with him. He whispered in my ear, "They are torturing me. Why would they do this to me?"

I could not answer, and that was the last question that he would ever ask me.

I made 13 trips to be with Jerry over the next year. At each visit, Jerry was worse and I was better. He never mentioned it, and I wondered what was going on in that brilliant mind of his. Did he wonder how it was possible that his little sister, with no knowledge of medicine, and without a Doctor, was actually getting better from Cancer with a protocol from American Indian Medicine Men and Women? I will never know, because he never spoke of it—but then he was so ill.

That year was the most difficult and the most glorious year of my life. Jerry and I loved each other deeply and dearly. He had so much love in his being, unlike any human I have ever known. It was a love of humanity; it included every one, and it included me. Jerry made his transition on February 18, 2013. He never complained; he never was irritated or in a bad mood toward the Doctors or Nurses. He respected everyone and always gave them his attention, and he made sure that they were honored.

Best of all, his children were by his side. Jerry loved them completely, and it was sheer joy for me to bask in his love for his children and grandchildren, my nieces and nephews, whom I love dearly. I want to be very sensitive that I do not say anything that would make them feel uncomfortable in any way.

Jerry was a very private person, and I will always do everything possible to honor him. I also know that in his new world, where he has a greater awareness of life, that he would want me to share with others the amazing miracle that I have found. He would want others to avoid the suffering and misery that he and our mom had endured, and I know he would Champion my cause of helping others with Cancer.

As I continue, then, with my story, I will tell you that I removed a total of 18 tumors from my right breast. This means that they simply fell out. At the end of two weeks, almost like clockwork, each tumor was released. After the 18th tumor, there were no more left. The wound simply closed up. There is a small scar, but that is a very little price to pay, isn't it? The tumors varied in size. The biggest one was the size of a silver dollar, with a depth of about 10 quarters, one on top of the other. This is layman's terms, but I did not know how to measure them with instruments.

I went to two Doctors for verification, and both Doctors witnessed the tumors, and I thought that I would have their testimonial for your consideration. One of them was a very well known Naturopathic Doctor in Scottsdale, Arizona, and the other was a very well-known MD and Homeopathic Doctor, also in Scottsdale. I was recently told by the office of the Naturopathic Doctor in Scottsdale that he cannot give me the testimonial because the Medical Board will not allow it. I am so grateful that Dr. Stanley Olsztyn had the courage to speak the truth, however, and you can read about his testimonial in Chapter 4.

Jerry had asked that I go to the Mayo Clinic in Phoenix, to their Breast Cancer Center, for additional tests of ultrasound and mammograms, just like the tests I had done at the Valley Radiologist in Phoenix. Both tests had showed I had a total of 3 tumors. So, I have to ask the question, why then were there 18 tumors that were released from my breast? The Doctors had no explanation, but maybe I do. Is it possible that the tumors travel to that point of the Two Feathers Healing Formula to be released? What other explanation could there be?

Each time a tumor fell out, there was also liquid that oozed from the wound. The tumors would have been much larger, if not for that fact. This suggests to me that tumors that may be in other areas of the body would also be liquefying and being released as waste in the body. I may not understand it all, but it does not matter whether I understand it. The body does understand, and it works with the herbal Two Feathers Healing Formula to return the body to health. At the same time, it is strengthening the immune system so that the body can fight any future Cancer.

I realize it is urgent and most important that I have an understanding of why I got the Cancer in the first place if I am to remain Cancer-free. That is why D. Gary Young, founder of Young Living Essential Oils, asks this question of any one who may have Cancer, "Why do you have Cancer?" Like many others, I do not know for sure, but I think it was the trauma of my life, both as a child and as an adult, that may be the root cause. It was also hereditary for me. Whatever the reasons were, I remain devoted to regaining my health.

I will continue with the Two Feathers Healing Formula, with a maintenance dose of one capsule daily. I have found, as I do an AMAS test every 3 months, that if I stop the regimen, my score begins to go back up. The AMAS test has a score of 0–700. Anything over 134 is considered to be Cancer. It is easy for me to keep my test score very low. If I see that the numbers are getting higher, I simply increase my dosage, but one capsule usually suffices. Therefore I have nothing to fear.

See my AMAS Oncology Test Scores in Chapter 5 and visit Oncolab's[9] website so that you can order the kit. It has to be done by a Doctor who has been trained to do it, and they will tell you about Doctors in your area who can do the test for you. The cost is about $400.00, and it is not covered by insurance. What a surprise.

People who choose conventional Cancer medicine do not have the AMAS test to help them to determine their Cancer, and how advanced it is. Doctors do not use it. Instead they use the PET Scan as a way to test for Cancer; however, the Mayo Clinic Doctor that I saw told me—and I quote—"Mayo Clinic does not use the PET Scan test because it actually causes Cancer. It has 300 times the Radiation of regular mammograms."

How disturbing this was for me to hear, as they were giving them to Jerry frequently, like giving out pancakes on a Sunday morning. My understanding is that they give sugar during the test, and since sugar feeds Cancer, then the sugar goes immediately to feed the Cancer, and they can track that. Why then do they not tell people that sugar feeds Cancer? There is another explanation why I had gotten Cancer. I was addicted to sugar. I thought that since I chose good sugar, like Agave or Maple Syrup that that would be ok. It wasn't ok for me because I already had Cancer and Candida, and I understand that now.

I use Stevia as my sweetener now. D. Gary Young speaks very strongly about the role that white sugar plays in Cancer, and especially in Candida, as a pre-cursor to Cancer. Please see Chapter 3 for my personal protocol using the Young Living Therapeutic Grade Essential Oils, Supplements, NingXia Red nutrient-rich drink, and the teachings of D. Gary Young in his *Essential Oils Desk Reference* guide.

I also gave up milk and cheese, along with the sugar, after studying the effects of eating these products.

There is another explanation for the possible reason I had this Cancer. I also have an Autoimmune Disease called Hashimoto's. It attacks my thyroid and is the cause of the chronic fatigue. Even though I have overcome the Cancer, I have not yet overcome the Hashimoto's. It makes sense to me that if I can overcome Cancer, then surely I can overcome an Autoimmune Disease. I continue to work on this, and even though I still have it, I have an amazing life. I can live with this, while I am determined to overcome it and have my Victory over Disease and Death.

I want to tell you that on this journey I have experienced several upsetting events. When my regular Doctor (and by that I mean the one that insurance covers—in my case, Medicare Insurance) realized that I was not going to have the Mastectomy, Radiation, and Chemo therapies, he dropped me. I was told not to come back until I had the surgery. He was extremely rude about it.

When I returned for the last test of the ultrasound and mammogram, I was told by the Radiologist to never return there either. He pointed his finger at me, and with a fierce rage, red face, and loud voice he said, "You are dying of Cancer! Never come back here again!" Then, he stuck his arm out at me, extending his hand, wanting me to shake it. How absurd that he would curse me using all of his power and authority to frighten me, to break my resolve, and then expect me to shake hands with him. How dare he do that to me! So, I wrote a letter to the Medical Board and complained about him. I received their answer. They replied, "He was perfectly within his rights to say what he said and do what he

Ha, I Laugh in the Face of Cancer

did." There was no justice for me here. I thank God that there will yet be Justice from Heaven.

I want to say that I have been shocked by the "Extreme Prejudice" I have encountered by Medical Doctors, Radiologists, Surgeons, and every health care professional that I have gone to for help, who have ridiculed me, threatened me to end medical assistance, and been most disrespectful to me when they learned I have overcome Cancer. Not one of them was interested in my success. They were, instead, angry and most agitated. The only exception to this was my personal Doctor, Dr. Stanley Olsztyn. He alone was sincerely happy for me, and he did not feel threatened but was thrilled that my life had been saved. Can you believe it?

Meanwhile, after a year, I am still Cancer-free. Too bad I can't go back and let him see my Victory! Maybe he will read my little book. While I am so grateful that I am Cancer-free, so many friends and acquaintances are not—in fact, they are all dead, except for a few whose Cancers are growing and spreading. I realize some people have overcome Cancer with conventional medicine. It just hasn't happened in my own personal experience. This has been such an incredible journey! Of course, I have tried to share with anyone who has come to me for help about my Two Feathers Healing Formula. I am shocked that no one was willing to commit to it in the way that I did.

One person who was referred to me chose, instead, to go to a very expensive Naturopathic Clinic in Europe. After 2 months, her tumors were bigger, and she returned home worse than before. She did try the Two Feathers Healing Formula at that time, but it was difficult because it is so important that you eat a hearty meal before using it. It is to be taken one hour after a good meal. She was so ill that it was hard to eat, and therefore, the Two Feathers Healing Formula nauseated her. I also was nauseated by it, but I wasn't as ill from the progression of the Cancer as she was. In the beginning I would feel ill, and I often vomited. But I learned that if I used my Young Living Peppermint Oil, it would help me. I also got an over-the-counter medication for nausea called Nausene. That also helped. As time went on, the nauseated feeling subsided, and I don't get it at all anymore. When someone is very ill, and the Cancer is spreading, they do have a problem. Best to catch it early, so be sure to do your preventative exams. Nevertheless, even in late-stage Cancer you can still have the same results that I have had, but the ride may be a little rougher. Don't give up! Be willing to try no matter how late in the game it is; remember, there can be a miracle for you, just like there was for me!

This precious lady continued the Two Feathers Healing Formula for some time before going once again to a Naturopathic Doctor who suggested she stop taking the Two Feathers Healing Formula. She obeyed and died a short time later. In her last surgery, her husband said the Doctor found evidence of dead Cancer that was probably the result of the Two Feathers Healing Formula.

Another dear friend of mine also had Breast Cancer. I sent her 2 bottles of the Two Feathers Healing Formula, and she was using it but not with the determination that is necessary for Victory. She went to see a Naturopathic Doctor who suggested she stop taking it. She listened, and since then the Cancer has progressed unchecked. It was in my opinion, a death sentence that Doctor had given her. There was nothing more that I could do.

Another person was referred to me, and I told her of my experience. She felt that her guidance was different and that as long as she did not believe the Cancer was real, it wasn't real. She would not speak the word or consider the reality. For me, it was important to speak the word, look at it, and deal with it. I believe in the power of the spoken word, but surely it must also include basic common sense and a protocol that works. Otherwise, the result is not that which is desired, to say the least. "Stand, Face, and Conquer"!

I have another dear friend that also was not interested in the Two Feathers Healing Formula. He went to healers, shamans, and practitioners of many wonderful modalities that he thought would work. He did many protocols of raw foods, cleansing, nutrients, wheatgrass—you name it, and he did it. I have never known anyone so devoted to his own healing! He went to very expensive Naturopathic Clinics and, after 5 months, he thinks that the Cancer is not growing, but he told me that he now has a feeding tube. He has not shared with me the results of his latest Medical Test. I can only hope that he will yet have his Victory! His Naturopathic Doctor had frightened him by saying that if the Two Feathers Healing Formula made the tumor in his throat come out, that that could kill him. This Doctor had no knowledge of the Two Feathers Healing Formula at all. But the damage had been done—Dr. God had spoken. My friend was afraid after that. My experience made it very clear that the tumors were actually melting each day that I looked at my wound, and the tumor material was actually pouring out. This means the tumors get smaller, absolutely! It occurred to me that if his tumor continued to grow, that would also kill him. I was so sorry to hear he had put his life's dream on hold, as his future is uncertain now. I do not understand his choice in view of the evidence of my experience. I have learned to be quiet and allow people their own choices, even though it is so painful for me to see the results of their programs.

The last example I have for you is a young mother with several children, who had a radical Mastectomy as well as Chemo treatments. Now, the Cancer has returned, and her Doctor has told her that she has stage 4 Cancer, and there is nothing left that can be done. I was so excited as a friend of a friend of this young mother called me, and I sent this person a copy of my book, and my offer to share with her my experience. I was sure that she would be willing to at least try to save her own life. However, she never responded to my offer. Perhaps she felt as if there was no real hope, because her Doctor had successfully influenced and convinced her that she was dying and nothing could be done. Like so many others I have known, she simply accepted her fate as determined by her Doctor, without even trying the Two Feathers Healing Formula. Her children will now grow up without their mother, and her husband will be without his wife.

It is necessary to make a brief statement here about a dear lady who was referred to me very late in her Cancer process. She had done it all, complying to every demand and suggestion of her Doctor. She had surgery, Chemo, and Radiation. In the END nothing had worked; the Cancer returned with a vengeance, her body could no longer tolerate additional Chemo, so her Doctor

Ha, I Laugh in the Face of Cancer

released her and she went to Hospice to live in what I know would be hell and misery. Just one more insult, however, because her Doctor suggested the "Peaceful" Pill, which I would more accurately call "The Suicide Pill." This death pill is legal in a few states, and Washington state where she lives is one of them. I guess her Doctor thought he was being "humane," to save her from what was yet to come. She agreed, and decided she would spend the Christmas Holidays with her family and take her Peaceful Pill after that. Is this humane, or is it an atrocity? You decide. I already know.

Just when you may think it can't get any worse than that, then consider this: "World News, headline, February 17, 2014, "Belgium approved child euthanasia" "Belgium's parliament has extended the right to die to terminally-ill children of all ages" What that means to me, is that most of the terminally ill children they are speaking of are young victims of Cancer, and the horrifying effects of Chemo and Radiation. If you are not outraged by this, then you must not have a heart that beats! What will happen to a world that allows parents and Doctors to kill the child who had no say in the treatment that brought the suffering in the first place? Do you want those consequences added to the already horrifying things that we continually do as a people?

I asked Robert Roy one time why the Doctors don't use the Two Feathers Healing Formula. He said it was too inexpensive to support their luxurious lifestyles and that Doctors are not required in the first place, as they are not needed for people to use the Two Feathers Healing Formula in their own healing. There you have it!

I found another reason also. The Naturopathic Doctor that

I went to for verification of my experience with the Two Feathers Healing Formula (taking photos of the tumors and watching them fall out) recognized immediately what I was doing. He took a photo of his brother out from his desk and showed me a picture of his brother who had a melanoma tumor right between his eyes. Then, he took out a specimen jar that had that very tumor in it! I was astounded that he knew all about the Two Feathers Healing Formula and had his own testimonial from his own brother.

So when I met several of his patients attending his Cancer clinic, he told me they were not doing well. They told me themselves they were not doing well. One had a radical Mastectomy, and lymph nodes removed, then later her female organs, and now the Cancer was back, and there were no more organs that could be removed. She was taking the intravenous treatments, but they were not helping. I had to ask the Doctor, "Why don't you tell them about the Two Feathers Healing Formula?" He said, "I can't! I know of one Doctor that gave it to his patient, and even though that patient was healed of Cancer; nevertheless, he almost lost his medical license for 'prescribing mud' to his patient." This moment will never be forgotten in my heart, because the consequences of this ignorance and arrogance of the Medical Review board will cost people their lives. Why?

While I was at this Naturopathic Cancer Clinic, I also had 10 intravenous, high potency Vitamin treatments. This was very expensive, and I borrowed $6,000.00 with a 25% interest rate from a credit card. Later, I questioned the wisdom of my choice when I realized that even if those 10 treatments had helped, it could not be continued because it was cost-prohibitive for me. It was not sustainable, and I had no way of determining whether it had even helped. Most disturbing was that I was left with a huge debt that, later, my beloved brother Jerry paid off in full for me.

If someone has huge sums of money and can invest in these expensive treatments, that is wonderful, but for most of us, that is just not going to work! I was encouraged when I saw a documentary about a new field of medicine called Naturopathic Oncology. I listened to it most intently and was quickly disappointed when I realized that the purpose of the good nutrition, which they called "Neutraceuticals," was to aid the body so that it could continue to take Chemo and Radiation when the body was too toxic to continue the deadly treatments. With the attention to nutrition, they "figured" that they could then pump more of the poison into the body. That is not what I had hoped for with this new Naturopathic Oncology. This new program will add huge sums of money to the already unbelievable amounts being placed upon the backs of the unsuspecting masses as they tread on with no reward of something that will really help. So get ready for Two Feathers Healing Formula, because I know it will REALLY help!

The $6,000.00 that I spent for intravenous vitamin/ nutrition therapy would have been better used for my own nutrition, purchasing fresh organic fruits, vegetables, seeds, and supplements. This use of my funds is wise because it is sustainable and something I need to do for the rest of my life. It is expensive, but I should have used my funds for this instead of 10 days of the intravenous vitamin/nutrition therapy.

What happens to patients who have become so toxic with

Chemo and Radiation that they can no longer continue to endure those treatments? Well, speaking from my own experience with my family members, the Doctors stop the treatments, and since the treatments have destroyed the body's own immune system, the Cancer spreads, unchecked of course.

It may be worse to continue the treatments, even if it kills the Cancer, because of the toxicity it creates in the body, because the suffering is so great. It sounds like a no-win situation to me.

It is also important to pose this question: why do the Oncology Doctors march mindlessly on, using toxic life-threatening treatments? It is as if they are blind, and deaf as well. They can't see, and they won't hear. They can't change their position, because how would that make them look? How will it look if they have been wrong all this time? They are so heavily indoctrinated that they have lost their ability to think clearly, or for themselves. They use their own medicine, so they must believe in it, but why? I am sorry, but it is a Zombie mentality. I don't mean to be disrespectful, but if they are disrespecting the truth and the evidence, and people are dying, then what else can be said?

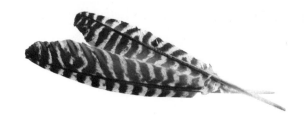

Chapter 2
This Is a "Do-It-Yourself Project"

I may not be able to help everyone, but surely there will be those who will recognize that my Victory can also be their Victory. This is a "do-it-yourself project"! It requires courage. The cost is so low that almost anyone—everyone—can afford it. If you want to try this for yourself, please contact Robert Roy at **www.healingformula.net** where you can purchase your Two Feathers Healing Formula. You may also email Robert Roy directly at **Robert@healingformula.net** or call him at **775-324-4889**. I am also available to help in every possible way, to encourage you to follow the regimen that worked for me. You can email me at **susan@hailaughinthefaceofcancer.com**.

Wouldn't it be a miracle if Cancer could be considered that kind of simple, but serious, illness that you could take care of from your own home, without an Oncology Doctor or Health Insurance, as I have done? Although this Protocol is simple, please never forget that Cancer is a life-threatening disease, and must always be treated with absolute caution. Of course it would require the type of determination and willingness to do your Two Feathers Healing

Formula Protocol as I have outlined for you here in this little book. The responsibility would be your own, the success would be determined by yourself, and the empowerment and Peace of Mind for winning your own health would be your greatest reward. Now, that would be a miracle!

It is also very important to me that I honor the American Indian Nations and their great Medicine Men and Women who have understood the miraculous healing ability of our Earth Mother. This honor will be different from the huge sums of money they get from Gambling Casinos. I am glad for their prosperity, but gambling causes such misery to others who are addicted, and those huge casinos everywhere, with the extravagant use of resources of electricity and water, are not good for our Earth Mother either. On the other hand, it is win-win for the Two Feathers Healing Formula, and no one loses. That is the kind of mercy and blessing that we all seek. "All for one and one for all."

I want to be very responsible with my little book. I also do not want to invoke the wrath of the Medical Community or any Entities that would like to hurt me, stop me, or cause me hardship. I have only one motive, and that is to be of service. If I can lessen someone's pain and suffering, if I can lighten someone else's burden, if I can ease their fear and nightmares, then that is what I will do. I ask to be protected by Angels and Heavenly Hosts.

Every book needs a Hero, and I have two of them! I would like to tell you about Robert Roy of Two Feathers Healing Formula. The Two Feathers Healing Formula has saved my life. Robert's assistance has been ever constant and helpful. He has never asked for one penny—NEVER! His devotion is absolute; his heart is pure, and I am humbled beyond words that I have been so blessed to have found him. He has helped over 60,000 people over a 30-year period! Let's all nominate him for one of those Heroes Awards they have on CNN Television!

My interest now is to protect and honor Robert Roy in our support for this Two Feathers Healing Formula through our prayers and actions. The Pharmaceutical Companies, the AMA, the FDA, and the tentacles of that giant mechanization monstrosity would stop at nothing to support their own Cancer Protocols. It is important to protect Robert—please remember that in your prayers. His courage to face this danger daily and help every one who seeks him out is a testimonial to his determination to help all people who suffer from Cancer and to help people like me to live and to thrive.

I am telling you about the most amazing miracle of my life, and I want to offer my little book and my testimonial to help others who may choose something other than conventional medicine, as I have. I am not prescribing. Let me repeat that, I AM NOT PRESCRIBING!!!! We must each be responsible for our own health care and health care decisions. When someone dies of Chemo or Surgery and complications that may arise, the Doctors are safe. They have insurance, they don't need to be afraid of a lawsuit, they are in no danger whatsoever. But Robert Roy flies by his Angel wings and knows that God will catch him if he falls. He is an honorable man, and I believe he is also a Holy man. He puts his life on the line every time he speaks to anyone who calls on him for help. That is what a Hero is to me.

I have a second Hero, who saved my life before I even got

Cancer in the first place. I am speaking about D. Gary Young, Founder of Young Living Essential Oils. When I was introduced to the Young Living Essential Oils, I was very ill and did not believe I could survive, physically, emotionally, or financially. But I began to use the oils in 1993, and I have been amazed at the healing in all aspects of my being. I told you earlier that I was too ill to work. That was true. The most miraculous journey began for me, and as I got well, I was also able to work, and my Young Living business as an Independent Distributor began to prosper and grow! Today, I have a very financially successful business that has sustained me for at least the last 15 years and will continue to do so for many years to come—in fact, I believe, for the rest of my life. When the economy failed so many people, my business continued to grow, because the oils are truly "Essential." The best part is that I love what I do, helping other people with their health and emotional issues with these amazing oils. I have written another book, dedicated to D. Gary and Mary Young and Young Living Oils, with a first-of-its-kind-ever scratch-and-sniff feature of our Essential Oils for children, called *Scented Adventures of The Bouquet Sisters in Fairyland.*[10]

There have been three extraordinary men in my life: my beloved brother Jerry, and then there was D. Gary Young, and, now, Robert Roy. So really, there are 3 Heroes in my little book!

If you would like to know more about my Protocol with my healing journey, please read Chapter 3 for more information about my life and Victory with Young Living Products. These oils are so essential to my life and well-being that I could never go even a day without them!

I would like to make mention here, of a very important

subject that is dear to my heart. It is the issue of our precious animal friends who have Cancer. Just as the Two Feathers Healing Formula works in people, so it also does the same work in animals. I had a most beloved Yellow Lab, named Sunshine. When I got Breast Cancer, at the same exact time, she also got Breast Cancer. I used the Two Feathers Healing Formula for her in a capsule at least once a day for a year, and her Vet said that he was amazed that I had kept her vibrant and well with this treatment. He said, "whatever you are doing please keep doing it!" Unfortunately, Sunshine passed into Spirit 3 months ago, but not of Cancer. She still had it, but it was on its way out. She died of old age at 15 and a half. That is a great miracle that I need to tell my readers.

Her Vet here in Phoenix is familiar with the Two Feathers Healing Formula, and she also uses it in her practice. She said that you have to be very careful, because one of her clients put the Two Feathers Healing Formula on her cat, without the assistance of this Vet. The Two Feathers Healing Formula was so strong, that it bore a whole through the cat's leg, and that was not good. Please be responsible when you are using this treatment. The Two Feathers Healing Formula can be used on tumors, and there are many examples and photos of before and after pictures of animals who have had amazing success. Just realize that you need to be aware. Please always check with Robert Roy about your pets.

I also have another animal story, about my beautiful Sable Sheltie, Jamie Girl. When Jamie was only 5 years old, I came home one day, and there was blood all over my bedroom where she had been. I was devastated, and put her on the bed to look her over. I could not see what might have been the cause, so of course I took her to her Vet the next day. The Vet said that Jamie Girl had tumors all over her tummy, and that the tumors were also growing on her in such a way that she could not go to the bathroom. He recommended that I take her home for the weekend, and bring her back on Monday to be put down.

I was heart sick, and I decided instead to do what I would have done if it were me that had those tumors (this was in 1994, before I had Cancer). So, I put her on the bed, and I looked in my Young Living *Essential Oils Desk Reference* Guide and followed the Protocol with the oils that I had that were on that list. I used Frankincense and Lavender, and I poured those two oils on her tummy. Then, I put her down off of the bed, she promptly went out the doggy door and went to the bathroom. There was no more blood! I used those oils on her daily after that. She lived a vibrant life for another 5 years with no issue of any kind. When it was time for her to leave me, to be born again in Spirit as a Puppy, I took her back to that same Vet. He looked at me and said, "Well she still has the tumors." I looked at him and said, "Yes, and I have had 5 fabulous years with her since you suggested we put her down." Why was he not happy and amazed that my Young Living Essential Oils had produced a miracle? Why indeed.

Since God has blessed me with such miracles as the Two Feathers Healing Formula and Young Living Essential Oils, they simply must be shared. I am thinking of you and offering to help. And of this you can be sure, "FIRST, I WILL DO NO HARM"!

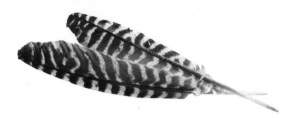

Chapter 3
Susan's Personal Regimen

Below is my regimen for my healing (am I allowed to say that word, or will I be arrested for speaking my truth?) from Cancer and preventative measures that I take to remain Cancer-free.

Two Feathers Healing Formula: You may contact Robert Roy at 775-324-4889 or visit his website at **www.healingformula.net**

Young Living Essential Oils and Supplements: Visit **www.ylwebsite.com/susanhall/home** (Susan Hall, Independent Distributor member number 9142). I use D. Gary Young's *Essential Oils Desk Reference* guide, which you can order at **www.lifesciencepublishers.com** or by calling 1-800-336-6308 (you can also purchase there my first book, *Scented Adventures of The Bouquet Sisters in Fairyland*). Look for his Cancer Protocol and teaching about Antioxidants, Inflammation, Immune System, Cleansing, and the Essential Oils and Supplements that are recommended.

- **Therapeutic Grade Essential Oils**
  - **Frankincense**—Item #3548
    Perhaps the most famous of all oils, used to increase spirituality and inner strength
  - **Myrtle**—Item #3596
    Supports respiratory function and thyroid health — also promotes uplifting and euphoric emotions
  - **Sandalwood**—Item #3634
    Promotes healthy, beautiful skin and encourages deeper meditation — also supportive of the body's natural defenses
  - **Tsuga**—Item #3352
    Has purifying properties and is spiritually uplifting

  These 4 oils are a protocol for breast cancer, so look at the book *Essential Oils Desk Reference* to see what is recommended by D. Gary Young for your particular situation.

- **NingXia Red Nutrient Rich Drink, 30 singles**—Item #3168
  Formulated to energize, fortify, and replenish the body and mind

- **ImmuPro Chewable Tablets**—Item #3213
  Formulated to enhance the immune system

- **Essentialzymes-4**—Item #4645
  A multi-spectral enzyme complex that aids the digestion of fats, proteins, fiber, and carbohydrates, allowing for optimal nutrient absorption

- **Valor**—Item #3429
  An empowering blend that promotes feelings of strength and courage

- **Joy**—Item #3372
  An uplifting blend of pure essential oils that creates magnetic energy and brings happiness to the heart

- **Peppermint**—Item #3614
  For digestion, mental and physical fatigue

- **Peace and Calming**—Item #3393
  This gentle scent encourages deep relaxation and can assist with meditation to promote a peaceful night's sleep

- **Sacred Mountain**—Item #3414
  A blend of Conifer and YlangYlang oils that evokes the sense of sanctity found in nature, and promotes feelings of self-strength, empowerment, grounding, and protection

- **Thyromin**—Item #3246
  A premium blend of bovine glandular extracts, herbs, amino acids, minerals, and oils to support a healthy Thyroid

- **Progessence Plus**—Item #4640
  A pure, harmonizing serum formulated specifically for women and designed to balance natural levels of progesterone in the body

- **Life 5 Probiotic**—Item #3099
  A high-potency probiotic that supports core intestinal health and promotes healthy immune function

- **Raindrop Technique**—Item #3137
  Designed to bring physical, emotional, and mental balance to the mind and body

If you wish to order these products, visit **www.ylwebsite.com/susanhall/home** (Susan Hall, Independent Distributor member number 9142), or call 800-371-3515 for Young Living Customer Service. Be sure to ask how to get the same wholesale prices that I get. If you would like my help, please email me at **susan@hailaughinthefaceofcancer.com**. Either I or my assistant will do everything possible to share with you what has worked for me.

Please remember, I can't prescribe anything, but I can tell you what I have done.

Exercise: Be sure to include exercise in your regimen. I use a good-quality minitrampoline. It only takes a few minutes a day, and be sure to pump your heels to cleanse the lymph system, as D. Gary Young taught me. If you are not steady on it, you can get one that has a stabilizing bar. Even if you do not jump, you can bounce. This will help to strengthen every atom of your being. Breathe deeply and use Aromatherapy to magnify your efforts.

Connect with Nature: Take your walk in soft moccasins, as the American Indians have done, and connect to the Earth Mother. Look at the beauty around you and the perfection of Nature. Take comfort in this. It is important to be at Peace in the midst of the Storm. Do your prayer or meditation, if that is your belief. Whatever your belief is, determine what makes you feel peaceful and use it. For me, it is the Young Living Essential Oil "Sacred Mountain."

Always Victory,

Susan Liberty Hall

Susan Liberty Hall

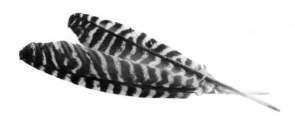

Chapter 4
Testimonials

I would like to introduce the testimonial of Dr. Stanley Olsztyn. Dr. Olsztyn is my Doctor, and he gives the AMAS tests to me that are so crucial for my accurate determination of the status of the Cancer. He also has helped me by simply observing in a most positive way, as I went through my Cancer Protocol with the Two Feathers Healing Formula. He was not afraid, like the other Doctors had been, that what I was doing might threaten him in some way because of my success. He was sincerely glad for my success. Isn't that what a Doctor should express? He had the courage to give me this testimonial when the other Doctor would not. He has earned his place as being "My Doctor," and I am very blessed to have him on my team.

> ❝ **Dr. Stanley Olsztyn's personal experience with Susan Hall and "Two Feathers Healing Formula"**
>
> Susan Hall first came to my office on June 20, 2012 to take a blood test called "AMAS" anti malignan antibody assay-which measures the body's immune system response to a protein produced ubiquitously by cancer cells. It was determined that she had breast cancer by her medical doctor, who had sent her to

have a mammogram, ultra sound, and biopsy of the area of concern. Cancer was found in two of the three biopsies that she had. She had found me through the AMAS Oncolab website as one of the Doctors in her area performing the AMAS testing.

The results of that test were "elevated", indicating that protein markers were in the problematic area and most probably produced by her right breast tumors. She told me she was using "Two Feathers Healing Formula" as her protocol to overcome this problem.

She continued to come to me regularly and about every three months she had another AMAS blood test to determine if her "Two Feathers Healing Formula" was successful in bringing down her test score. The second blood test was on August 28, 2012, and this test had a net tag score of 42. This is considered to be in the normal range and is in fact very low normal, the lower the test score the better.

She felt that this was the evidence that she needed to feel that the breast cancer was no longer growing or spreading. On examinations I was able to see the tumors and their being extruded from the breast. She asked me for specimen jars and preservative to keep the tumors in.

On January 24, 2013, her test score was 16, indicating that not only was it normal, but it was one of the lowest scores I had seen in 25 years of testing.

The next test was November 29, 2012 with a

test score of 91. This score was in the "Normal" range as any score under 134 is considered to be "Normal". Any score over 134 is considered to be "Elevated". With the score going up, she told me that she increased her dosage of the "Two Feathers Healing Formula". In this way, she felt that she could better control the cancer.

On May 23, 2013, her test score was at 130, indicating "Borderline". Susan had stopped taking the "Two Feathers Healing Formula" for the last several months, and now felt that she needed to go back on a good maintenance dosage.

On August 20, 2013, her test score was 32, indicating that she was once again in the low "Normal" test range. She was very relieved, and confident that she was well and that a maintenance program of the "Two Feathers" would keep her well.

I saw the tumors that had been extruded from her right breast. It was a heart warming experience for me to accompany Susan on her journey to recover. I will continue to see her and to repeat periodic AMAS testings. **"**

Stanley R. Olsztyn M.D.H.

Doctor Olsztyn is co-founder and past President of the Arizona Homeopathic Medical Association. As a Ford Foundation Merit Scholar, he attended undergraduate school at Marquette University in Milwaukee, Wisconsin and Medical College at Wayne State University in Detroit, Michigan. After post graduate training in Baltimore, he was certified by the American Board of Psychiatry and Neurology.

He has served as Examiner, Consultant and Instructor in Psychiatry. For two years, he was Chief of Neuropsychiatry at Hunter Air Force Base in Savannah, Georgia. For three years he was coordinator of a Pain and Stress Control clinic in Cleveland, Ohio during which time he was a visiting lecturer at the Cleveland Clinics in Ohio.

With three other well known and respected Medical Doctors, he helped establish the first fully accredited Residency Training Program in Psychiatry at Samaritan Health Services in Phoenix, Arizona. He was in charge of Intern Training in Psychiatry and lectured extensively in areas of pain management, stress, hypnosis and body-mind-emotional interactions in health and illness.

Over the years Doctor Olsztyn spent time training at various prestigious American medical centers, hospitals and clinics, studying with world renown allergists, immunologists, endocrinologists and metabologists. Many months were spent in Europe and Mexico learning from physicians whose patients were a Who's Who of world statesman, artists, actors and Religious Leaders.

Doctor Olsztyn now practices in Phoenix, Arizona and has incorporated into his general practice the latest proven techniques of conventional and alternative medicine. He recently received his Medical University's Distinguished Service Award for twenty five years of outstanding medical service to his communities.

STANLEY R. OLSZTYN, M.D.(H.), P.C.
PREVENTIVE MEDICINE
8580 E. Shea Blvd., Suite 110
Scottsdale, Arizona 85260
Phone (480) 948-0500
Fax (480) 948-0533
HealingAmericaMedicalClinic.com
HealingTheWorld.org
IMMUNIZEOLOGY.COM
IMMUNIZEOLOGYPets.com

I just heard from another Doctor, Dr. Sarah Kalomiros, D.C. of Kalo Clinic Natural Health and Healing Center[11] in San Francisco, who just referred one of her Stage 4 Cancer patients to me to do the Two Feathers Healing Formula.

So, here is a second Doctor, in addition to Dr. Olsztyn, that is not only open to, but willing to refer patients to Robert Roy.

Please read the following amazing testimonial of the first of many who will declare, "Ha, I Laugh in the Face of Cancer."

66 Hi Susan,

My name is Patricia ... I have sent you a Friend Request and message on Facebook, and wanted to reach out to you here as well since you were so kind to include your email address in your story on Robert's FB Page... which btw I LOVE your domain page!!! It's absolutely perfect!!!

I would love any further information you might share about your experience in using the Two Feathers formula... I have been using it for a month or so and have just had my first tumor area fall off!!! OMG what an exciting experience this is!!!

I was relieved to read in your story that your hole left by the tumor extraction eventually healed itself and would appreciate any advice you can share so that I too might have the same outcome in my future!!!

With much gratitude for your sharing your story and your offer to help those of us who are following in your footsteps :)))

I too am now laughing in the face of cancer!!!! 99

—Patricia

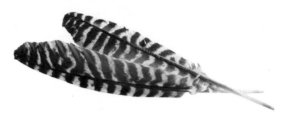

Chapter 5
Susan's AMAS Test Scores

Dear Readers,

The following are my actual AMAS test results for your review. Please look at the Net Tag column of the Component Results for the score. Any score under 134 is considered normal. I feel it is very relevant to explain the importance of using the AMAS blood test as a way to help you to have your Victory over Cancer. I suggest getting one as soon as possible so that you have a way of knowing your score, and then watch it go down as you continue with the Two Feathers Healing Formula.

When you can see your success, this will encourage you to continue and to be determined to not give up until you are Cancer-free. You can then continue the tests every 3 months as well to be sure you remain Cancer-free. I did not listen to Robert Roy when he told me to continue a maintenance dose, after I received a very low score on the test of 16 (see AMAS test result number 130107). It was the lowest score my Homeopathic Doctor had ever seen, and I was very confident that I was Cancer-free. Robert Roy said to be very sure the Cancer was completely gone before I stopped taking the Two Feathers Healing Formula; however, 3 months later, my score had gone up to 130! This was still not Cancer, but it was borderline. I learned my lesson, and now I listen to everything that Robert Roy suggests for my success.

The score of 150 (See AMAS test result number 120948) shows an elevated score, indicating I had Cancer. That was the first AMAS test that I had, and I had already been on the Two Feathers Healing Formula for several months. If I had taken the test when I first knew I had Cancer, several months before, it would probably have been much higher than 150. I regret I did not have it immediately upon realizing I had Cancer. I am certain that it had come way down (to 150) by the time I had been doing the regimen for several months.

It is very important to have a way to determine that what you are doing is working for you. The AMAS test is imperative for this understanding. This is the diagnostic tool that I must have for my peace of mind.

Results of AMAS® DETERMINATION
(Anti-Malignin Antibody in Serum, determined with Target® Reagent)

Oncolab
36 Fenway, Boston, MA 02215
p (617) 536-0850 f (617) 536-0657
www.oncolabinc.com

130998

Physician's Name: Olsztyn, Stanley

Patient's Name: Hall, Susan, DOB 5/28/1945

Lab Director: Samuel Bogoch, M.D., Ph.D   Technician: Blaszkiewicz, Magda

Fax Number: (480) 948-0533

Determination Date: 8/20/2013

Component Results

AMA ug/m	S-TAG	F-TAG	Net TAG
700-			
500-699			
400-499			
300-399			
135-299	156		
100-134		124	
25-99			32
0-24			

Overall Result

☐	**ELEVATED** Confirmatory repeat test recommended
☐	**BORDERLINE** Confirmatory repeat test recommended
X	**NORMAL** Can also occur in successfully treated cancer patients with "no evidence of disease" and in advanced or terminal patients with antibody failure
☐	**INCONCLUSIVE** Duplicates do not aree, or laboratory error: please repeat at Oncolab's expense

---

Results of AMAS® DETERMINATION
(Anti-Malignin Antibody in Serum, determined with Target® Reagent)

Oncolab
36 Fenway, Boston, MA 02215
p (617) 536-0850 f (617) 536-0657
www.oncolabinc.com

130635

Physician's Name: Olsztyn, Stanley

Patient's Name: Hall, Susan, DOB 5/28/1945

Lab Director: Samuel Bogoch, M.D., Ph.D   Technician: Blaszkiewicz, Magda

Fax Number: (480) 948-0533

Determination Date: 5/23/2013

Component Results

AMA ug/m	S-TAG	F-TAG	Net TAG
700-			
500-699			
400-499			
300-399			
135-299	252		
100-134		122	130
25-99			
0-24			

Overall Result

☐	**ELEVATED** Confirmatory repeat test recommended
X	**BORDERLINE** Confirmatory repeat test recommended
☐	**NORMAL** Can also occur in successfully treated cancer patients with "no evidence of disease" and in advanced or terminal patients with antibody failure
☐	**INCONCLUSIVE** Duplicates do not aree, or laboratory error: please repeat at Oncolab's expense

---

Ha, I Laugh in the Face of Cancer

Oncolab

Results of AMAS® DETERMINATION
(Anti-Malignin Antibody in Serum, determined with Target® Reagent)

36 Fenway, Boston, MA 02215
p (617) 536-0850 f (617) 536-0657
www.oncolabinc.com

130107

Physician's Name: Olsztyn, Stanley

Patient's Name: Hall, Susan, DOB 5/28/1945

Lab Director: Samuel Bogoch, M.D., Ph.D Technician: Blaszkiewicz, Magda

Fax Number: (480) 948-0533

Determination Date: 2/24/2013

Component Results

AMA ug/m	S-TAG	F-TAG	Net TAG
700-			
500-699			
400-499			
300-399			
135-299	140		
100-134		124	
25-99			
0-24			16

Overall Result

☐ **ELEVATED**
Confirmatory repeat test recommended

☐ **BORDERLINE**
Confirmatory repeat test recommended

☒ **NORMAL**
Can also occur in successfully treated cancer patients with "no evidence of disease" and in advanced or terminal patients with antibody failure

☐ **INCONCLUSIVE**
Duplicates do not aree, or laboratory error: please repeat at Oncolab's expense

---

Oncolab

Results of AMAS® DETERMINATION
(Anti-Malignin Antibody in Serum, determined with Target® Reagent)

36 Fenway, Boston, MA 02215
p (617) 536-0850 f (617) 536-0657
www.oncolabinc.com

121760

Physician's Name: Olsztyn, Stanley

Patient's Name: Hall, Susan, DOB 5/28/1945

Lab Director: Samuel Bogoch, M.D., Ph.D Technician: Blaszkiewicz, Magda

Fax Number: (480) 948-0533

Determination Date: 11/29/2012

Component Results

AMA ug/m	S-TAG	F-TAG	Net TAG
700-			
500-699			
400-499			
300-399			
135-299	167		
100-134			
25-99		76	91
0-24			

Overall Result

☐ **ELEVATED**
Confirmatory repeat test recommended

☐ **BORDERLINE**
Confirmatory repeat test recommended

☒ **NORMAL**
Can also occur in successfully treated cancer patients with "no evidence of disease" and in advanced or terminal patients with antibody failure

☐ **INCONCLUSIVE**
Duplicates do not aree, or laboratory error: please repeat at Oncolab's expense

Ha, I Laugh in the Face of Cancer

Results of AMAS® DETERMINATION
(Anti-Malignin Antibody in Serum, determined with Target® Reagent)

Oncolab
36 Fenway, Boston, MA 02215
p (617) 536-0850 f (617) 536-0657
www.oncolabinc.com

121305

Physician's Name: Olsztyn, Stanley

Patient's Name: Hall, Susan

Lab Director: Samuel Bogoch, M.D., Ph.D

Fax Number: (480) 948-0533

Determination Date: 8/28/2012

Technician: Blaszkiewicz, Magda

Component Results

AMA ug/m	S-TAG	F-TAG	Net TAG
700-			
500-699			
400-499			
300-399			
135-299	184	142	
100-134			
25-99			42
0-24			

Overall Result

☐	**ELEVATED** Confirmatory repeat test recommended
☐	**BORDERLINE** Confirmatory repeat test recommended
X	**NORMAL** Can also occur in successfully treated cancer patients with "no evidence of disease" and in advanced or terminal patients with antibody failure
☐	**INCONCLUSIVE** Duplicates do not aree, or laboratory error: please repeat at Oncolab's expense

---

Results of AMAS® DETERMINATION
(Anti-Malignin Antibody in Serum, determined with Target® Reagent)

Oncolab
36 Fenway, Boston, MA 02215
p (617) 536-0850 f (617) 536-0657
www.oncolabinc.com

120948

Physician's Name: Olsztyn, Stanley

Patient's Name: Hall, Susan

Lab Director: Samuel Bogoch, M.D., Ph.D

Fax Number: (480) 948-0533

Determination Date: 6/20/2012

Technician: Walsh, Kevin

Component Results

AMA ug/m	S-TAG	F-TAG	Net TAG
700-			
500-699			
400-499			
300-399			
135-299	279		150
100-134		129	
25-99			
0-24			

Overall Result

X	**ELEVATED** Confirmatory repeat test recommended
☐	**BORDERLINE** Confirmatory repeat test recommended
☐	**NORMAL** Can also occur in successfully treated cancer patients with "no evidence of disease" and in advanced or terminal patients with antibody failure
☐	**INCONCLUSIVE** Duplicates do not aree, or laboratory error: please repeat at Oncolab's expense

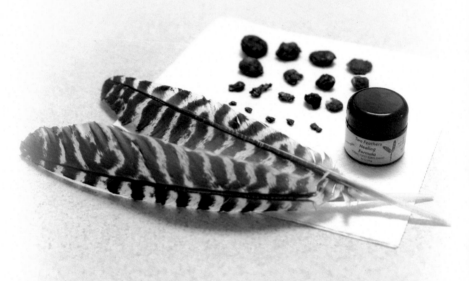

18 Tumors,
Dead and Gone

The dark color of the tumors is the residue of the
Two Feathers Healing Formula that they were
preserved in this last year and a half.
The original color was a grayish-white color,
like a fungus might be.

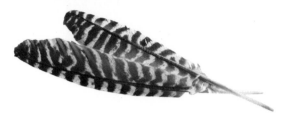

Chapter 6
Cancer Statistics

I am including this chapter and some facts and figures[12] for your consideration as we all ponder the devastation of Cancer. This is just the tip of the iceberg, and it is staggering and astounding when you begin to understand what the consequences are for us to continue down the road of failure. Time to take the road less traveled.

Economic Impact of Cancer: The financial costs of Cancer are high for both the person with Cancer and for society as a whole. The National Institutes of Health (NIH) estimated the 2012 overall annual costs of Cancer were as follows:

- **Total Cost:** $201.5 billion
- **Direct Medical Costs:** $77.4 billion (total of all health expenditures)
- **Indirect Mortality Costs:** $124 billion (cost of lost productivity due to premature death)
- One of the major costs of Cancer is Cancer treatments. But lack of health insurance and other barriers to health care prevent many Americans from even getting good, basic health care.

According to the US Census Bureau, about 50 million people were uninsured in 2012 and about 10% of children in the United States had no health insurance coverage in 2012.

This year (2013), about 580,350 US Residents are expected to die from Cancer. That is nearly 1,600 people a day.

Cancer is the second most common cause of death in the United States, exceeded only by heart disease. Medical error is the third leading cause of death[13]. I have a personal experience regarding medical error, as my son's beloved grandfather died at a young age, from a simple test in the hospital, that would be understood as Medical Error, but just try to prove it!

Cancer accounts for nearly 1 out of every 4 deaths in the United States.

Cancer costs billions of dollars. It also costs us the people we love. Reducing barriers to Cancer care is critical in the fight to eliminate suffering and death due to Cancer.

Based on rates from 2007–2009, 12.38% of women born today will be diagnosed with Cancer of the breast at some time during their lifetime. This number can also be expressed as 1 in 8 women will be diagnosed with Cancer of the breast during their lifetime.

It is estimated that 232,340 women will be diagnosed with, and 39,620 women will die, of Cancer of the breast in 2013.

Ha, I Laugh in the Face of Cancer

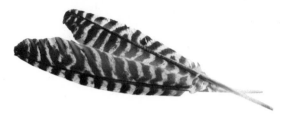

References and Other Resources

[1]Hulda Clark, *The Cure for All Cancers*
www.huldaclark.com

[2]David Icke, "Cancer Is a Fungus—and It Is Curable"
www.davidicke.com

[3]Tullio Simoncini
www.curenaturalicancro.com

[4]Jim Humble, *The Miracle Mineral Solution of the 21st Century*
jhbooks.org/the-miracle-mineral-solution-of-the-21st-century

[5]Jim Humble, Sodium Chlorite Water Purification Drops
www.BetterWPD.com

[6]Two Feathers Healing Formula
www.healingformula.net

[7]Young Living Essential Oils
www.ylwebsite.com/susanhall/home

[8]NovaVita Clinic
Phone: 011-593-4288-3480
Email: *novavitaresearchcenter@hotmail.com*

[9]AMAS by Oncolab
www.oncolabinc.com

[10]*Scented Adventures of The Bouquet Sisters in Fairyland*
www.thebouquetsisters.com

[11]Dr. Sarah Kalomiros, D.C.
www.kaloclinic.com

[12]American Cancer Society, Cancer Facts & Figures 2013
www.cancer.org/research/cancerfactsfigures/cancerfactsfigures/
cancer-facts-figures-2013

[13]Health Impact News Daily, "Death of Americans: The Medical System is Now the Third Leading Cause of Death in the U.S."
www.healthimpactnews.com/2013/death-of-americans-the-medical-system-is-now-the-third-leading-cause-of-death-in-the-u-s/

Other Resources

Global Healing Center, "The Truth About Cancer..."
www.globalhealingcenter.com/truth-about-cancer/the-truth-about-cancer

Global Healing Center, "Facts You Need to Know About Cancer"
www.globalhealingcenter.com/truth-about-cancer/facts-you-need-to-know-about-cancer

Global Healing Center, "Chemotherapy Quotes"
www.globalhealingcenter.com/truth-about-cancer/chemotherapy-quotes

Disclaimer and Reader Agreement

The writings, thoughts, and views expressed in Ha, I Laugh in the Face of Cancer are solely those of the author and do not necessarily represent those of any other third party listed in this book. Ha, I Laugh in the Face of Cancer is not endorsed by or affiliated with any of these third parties.

Under no circumstances will the author or publisher be liable to any person or business entity for any direct, indirect, special, incidental, consequential, or other damages based on any use of this book or any other source to which it refers, including, without limitation, any lost profits, business interruption, or loss of programs or information.

The author is not a medical doctor. It is wise at all times to consult a licensed medical doctor, naturopath, or health professional for any type of health issue. The information presented here is not intended to be a prescription or substitute for professional health care. The author has found allopathic doctors to be very helpful with diagnosis, emergency care, and necessary surgery.

By reading this book, you, the reader, consent to bear sole responsibility for your own decisions to use or read any of this book's material. Neither the author nor the publisher shall be liable for any damages or costs of any type arising out of any action taken by you or others based upon reliance on any materials in this book.

Note About Therapeutic Grade Essential Oils

Please be advised that the Therapeutic Grade Essential Oils spoken of in this book are very strong medicines, so please use caution when you use your oils. Susan Liberty Hall and her assistants would be happy to teach you about the oils, and they have literature and CDs to help you learn about them. If you wish to have more information, please contact Susan at susan@hailaughinthefaceofcancer.com or visit her website at www.ylwebsite.com/susanhall/home.

Website Links and References

All website links referenced in this book are current as of the publication of this book, December 2013.

I would like to thank Bob Anderson for copy editing the manuscript.

I would also like to thank Monica Stanley for the beautiful photographs in this book. www.monicastanleyphotography.com

Nick Ligidakis, the best publisher in the world, www.Inkwellproductions.com

Lilly Skye, for her fabulous book design, and art work, www.studioskye.com

Dea Shandera, for her amazing work as my Media Consultant.
deashandera@gmail.com

Brandon Hall, my son, and Computer consultant, and the best Realtor in Arizon
www.inhabitrealtyaz.com

My "Company of Angels" Young Living leaders and their devotion and support
www.ylwebsite.com/susanhall

and especially, Maureen Agganis, my personal Assistant, and dearest friend and
loyal supporter, "Way to grow lawn Service", Phoenix Az.
waytogrowlawnservice@yahoo.com

"Pray for the Cure"   www.prayforthecure.info